CW00508179

Low Carbs Cocktails

A Collection of Tasty Keto Friendly Alcohol Drinks Recipes from Ketogenic Margarita to Low Carbs Negroni and Old Fashioned

Jenny Kern

Table Of Contents

Introduction

Thank you for purchasing this book. In recent years, the culture of drinking has considerably evolved and cocktail enthusiasts have rapidly increased not only in number, but also and above all in the awareness of a conscious consumer to safeguard their palate and health. With this book you will learn how to make your favorite cocktails that you can enjoy alone or in company. What are you waiting for to enter the world of cocktails and make a great figure! Hope you can get passionate and become a true master.

Enjoy.

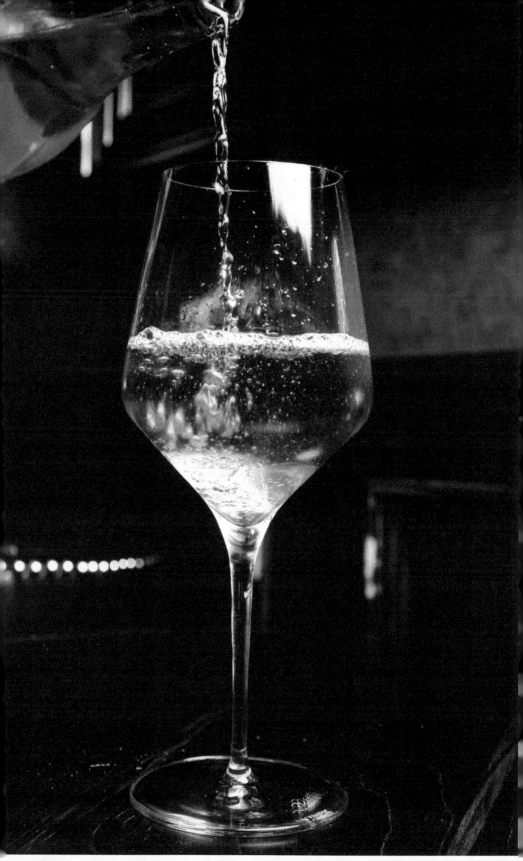

Wine and Champagne Keto Cocktails

Spanish Sparkling Cocktail

Preparation time: 10 minutes

Servings: 7

Ingredients:

Distilled water

10 clementines

½ c. sugar

1 ½ c. amontillado sherry

1 ½ c. Spanish brandy

Whole nutmeg

1 ½ cup cava or Spanish sparkling wine, chilled

Directions:

Peel two of the clementines, then separate them into segments. Fill a quart-sized container or Bundt pan with the distilled water and add in the segmented clementines to produce decorative ice blocks.

Peel the 8 remaining clementines. Mix sugar and the clementine peels in a bowl. Use a wooden spoon to muddle the peel and the sugar mixture. Continue until you notice that the oils from the clementine peels infuse into the sugar. Set the mixture aside for a minimum of ninety minutes at room temperature.

Juice the clementines until you get one cup of juice from them. Pour this juice into the sugar and peels mix. Stir the mixture until all the sugar is dissolved. Use a sieve to strain the liquid and add it to a punch bowl. Remove all the peels.

Add sherry to the bowl then pour in the brandy. Stir the mixture well.

Once done, you can unmold the ice block. Gently place it into the bowl. Add in the cava then stir the mixture gently.

Add a bit of grated nutmeg on top of the punch.

Strawberry Champagne

Preparation time: 10 minutes

Servings: 2

Ingredients:

12 ounces champagne

1 12-oz. can limeade concentrate, frozen

8 ounces tequila

12 ounces water

4 ounces strawberry liquor

Directions:

Put some ice into the pitcher then pour the limeade over it. Fill the limeade can with champagne. Make sure that the can is full and pour it into the pitcher.

Next, fill the can with tequila and strawberry liquor. Add this mixture into the pitcher.

Add water to the pitcher. Stir the mixture well. Serve with ice.

Juicy Fruit Champagne

Preparation time: 10 minutes

Servings: 2

Ingredients:

2 tbsps. pineapple juice

4 fluid-ounces orange juice

2 fluid-ounces carbonated beverage with lemon-lime flavor

4 fluid-ounces cranberry juice

¼ c. strawberries, sliced and frozen

2 fluid-ounces champagne

2 fluid-ounces apple juice

Directions:

Mix cranberry, pineapple, apple, and orange juice in a pitcher or bowl.

Add the carbonated beverage, sliced strawberries, and champagne. Let the mixture set for around 1-2 minutes to allow the strawberries to thaw.

Pour the drink into glasses then serve.

Mulled Apple Champagne Punch

Preparation time: 10 minutes

Servings: 15

Ingredients:

1 tbsp. orange zest, grated

3 tbsps. pumpkin pie spice

1 12-fluid oz. can apple juice concentrate, frozen then thawed

1 8-oz. can pineapple chunks

3-qt. Chablis wine

1 750-ml. bottle dry champagne, chill before using

1 4-oz. jar drained maraschino cherries

1 orange, slice them into round shapes

Directions:

Mix orange zest, pumpkin pie spice, and apple juice concentrate in a pan. Boil the mixture then simmer for around ten minutes. Once done, you can remove the pan from heat. Add white wine. Store in the fridge to chill overnight.

Use a coffee filter to strain the chilled wine mix. Be careful to avoid disturbing the spices that have already settled at the bottom part of the pitcher.

To prepare the ice ring, you just need to mix the maraschino cherries, orange slices, and pineapple chunks in a mold shaped like a ring. Fill the rest of the mold with water. Freeze overnight.

Unmold the ice ring, slice into pieces and add it to the punch

White Wine Citrus Sangria

Preparation time: 5 minutes

Servings: 8

Ingredients:

1 sliced navel orange, large

2 sliced lemons, fresh

2 sliced limes, fresh

1/4 cup of mint leaves, fresh

1/2 cup of vodka, citrus

2 tbsp. of nectar, agave

2 bottles of wine, dry white

Directions:

Add all ingredients to a large-sized pitcher.

Stir to combine well.

Add ice to glasses and serve.

Berry Wine Cocktail

Preparation time: 10 minutes

Servings: 2

Ingredients:

1 cup dry white wine

½ oz crème de cassis

½ cup raspberries

Directions:

Pour créme de cassis equally into each glass.

Pour white wine on top and top with raspberries.

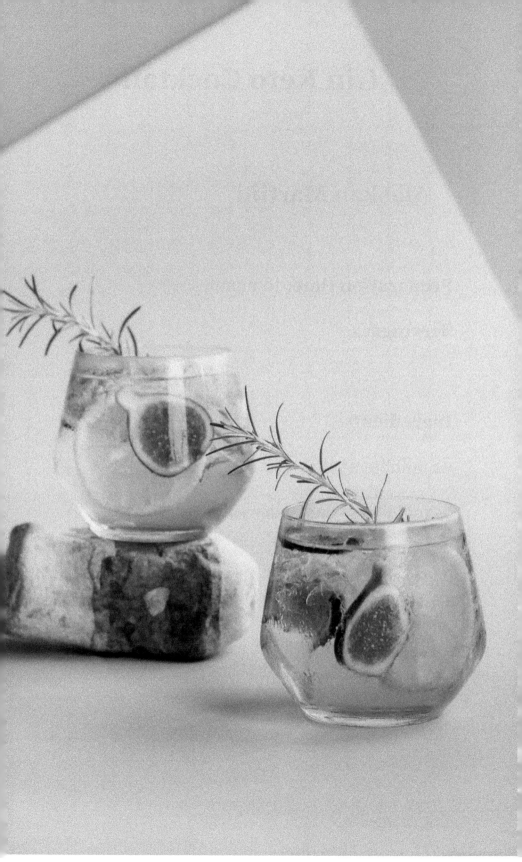

Gin Keto Cocktails

Alaskan Martini

Preparation time: 10 minutes

Servings: 2

Ingredients:

22 milliliters yellow Chartreuse

75 milliliters London dry gin

Directions:

Stir all ingredients with ice and strain into chilled glass. Garnish using mint.

Corpse Reviver

Preparation time: 10 minutes

Servings: 2

Ingredients:

4 milliliters absinthe

22 milliliters lemon juice

22 milliliters Lillet Blanc

22 milliliters London dry gin

22 milliliters triple sec

Directions:

Shake ingredients with ice and strain into chilled glass. Garnish using lemon zest twist.

Gin Star

Preparation time: 10 minutes

Servings: 2

Ingredients:

8 milliliters sugar syrup

15 milliliters lime juice

60 milliliters gin

top with soda

Directions:

Shake the first three ingredients with ice and strain into ice-filled glass. Top with soda. Garnish with lime zest twist.

Gin Salad Dry Martini

Preparation time: 10 minutes

Servings: 2

Ingredients:

15 milliliters dry vermouth

1 dash orange bitters

75 milliliters London dry gin

Directions:

Stir ingredients with ice and strain into chilled glass. Garnish using green olives and cocktail onions.

Gin Blast

Preparation time: 10 minutes

Servings: 2

Ingredients:

15 milliliters lemon juice

30 milliliters elderflower liqueur

2 dashes lemon bitters

60 milliliters London dry gin

3 fresh basil leaves

top with tonic water

Directions:

Lightly muddle (just to bruise) basil in the base of the shaker. Put in other ingredients except for tonic, shake with ice, and strain into ice-filled glass. Top with tonic water. Garnish using lemon zest twist.

Gibson Dry Martini

Preparation time: 10 minutes

Servings: 2

Ingredients:

15 milliliters dry vermouth

75 milliliters London dry gin

Directions:

Stir ingredients with ice and strain into chilled glass. Garnish using two cocktail onions.

Rosé black tea

Preparation time: 60 minutes

Servings: 4

Ingredients:

2 sachets of orange-flavored black tea

1 orange

ice cubes

2 cups of boiling water

1 cup of Martini Rosé

orange peel to decorate

Directions:

Heat the water until it is boiling and soak the tea bags for 5 minutes. Leave to cool, then put to cool in the refrigerator for about an hour.

Meanwhile, with a pestle, pound the orange cut into small pieces in 4 glasses. Add the iced tea and divide Martini Rosé.

Stir, then add 3 ice cubes to each glass, garnish with orange zest and serve.

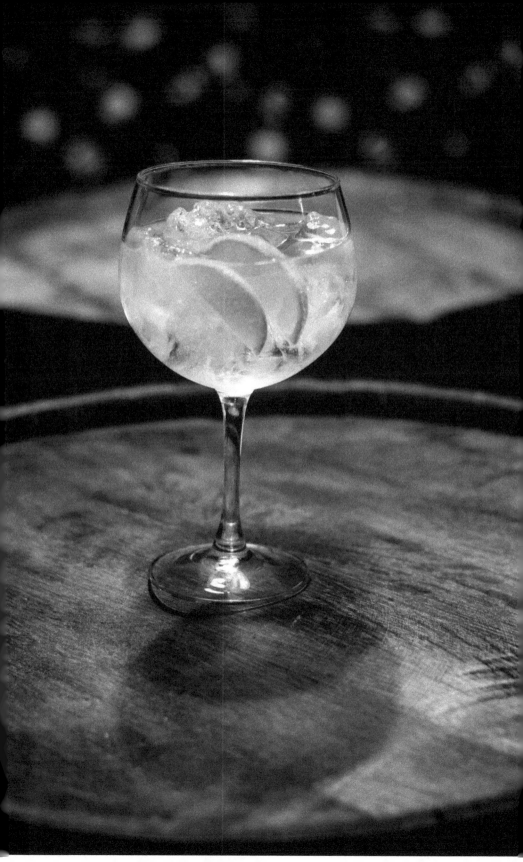

Whiskey Keto Cocktails

New York Flip

Preparation time: 10 minutes

Servings: 2

Ingredients:

15 milliliters sugar syrup

15 milliliters tawny port

1 fresh egg (white and yolk)

45 milliliters bourbon whiskey

Directions:

Vigorously shake ingredients with ice and strain into chilled glass. Garnish using grated nutmeg.

New York Cocktail

Preparation time: 10 minutes

Servings: 2

Ingredients:

22 milliliters apple schnapps liqueur

22 milliliters sweet vermouth

1 dash whiskey barrel-aged bitters

45 milliliters bourbon whiskey

Directions:

Stir ingredients with ice and strain into chilled glass.
Garnish using maraschino cherry.

Mountain Raze

Preparation time: 10 minutes

Servings: 2

Ingredients:

8 milliliters falernum liqueur

30 milliliters cranberry juice

30 milliliters pink grapefruit juice

1 teaspoon runny honey

45 milliliters bourbon whiskey

Directions:

Stir honey with bourbon in the base of the shaker to dissolve honey. Put in other ingredients, shake with ice, and strain into chilled glass. Garnish using grapefruit zest twist.

Mississippi Punch

Preparation time: 10 minutes

Servings: 2

Ingredients:

22 milliliters Cognac V.S.O.P.

22 milliliters lemon juice

30 milliliters sugar syrup

45 milliliters bourbon whiskey

60 milliliters cold water

Directions:

Shake ingredients with ice and strain into a glass filled with crushed ice. Garnish using a lemon slice.

Mint Julep

Preparation time: 10 minutes

Servings: 2

Ingredients:

22 milliliters sugar syrup

12 fresh mint leaves

75 milliliters bourbon whiskey

3 dashes bitters

Directions:

Shake ingredients with ice, strain into a julep cup filled with crushed ice, and stir. Garnish using lemon slices and mint dusted with confectioner's sugar.

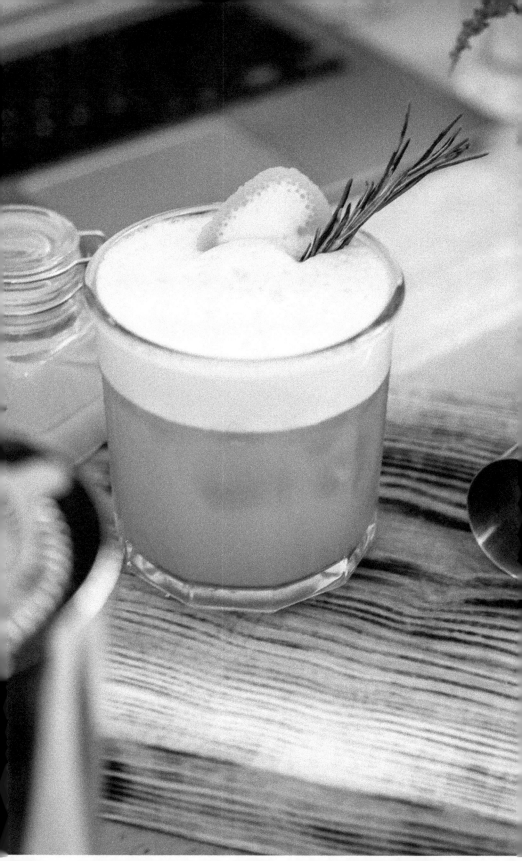

Tequila Cocktails

Tequila Sunrise

Preparation time: 10 minutes

Servings: 2

Ingredients:

50 ml (1.7 oz.) tequila

2 tbsp grenadine

1 tbsp triple sec

Ice cubes

The juice of 1 orange

The juice of ½ lemon

1 cocktail cherry

Directions:

Place the grenadine into the base of one tall glass.

Put the triple sec, tequila, fruit juices, and ice into a cocktail shaker and shake well.

Add ice cubes to the tall glass and then double strain your cocktail into it.

Serve with additional ice and garnish with a cherry on a cocktail stick.

Duke Tulip

Preparation time: 10 minutes

Servings: 2

Ingredients:

1½ oz. gold tequila

½ oz. vanilla syrup

½ oz. sugar syrup

Lemon

Orange

Raspberry

Rosemary

Ice

Directions:

Place a quarter of lemon, 2 orange wedges, a rosemary sprig into a shaker and muddle

Pour in ½ oz. of sugar syrup, ½ oz. of vanilla syrup, and 1½ oz. of gold tequila

Fill the shaker with ice cubes and shake

Finely strain into a chilled champagne saucer

Garnish with 2 raspberries on a rosemary sprig

Frozen blueberry margaritas

Preparation time: 10 minutes

Servings: 2

Ingredients:

2ml Blanco tequila

½ cup ice cubes

1 ½ ml fresh orange juice

½ cup frozen blueberries

2teaspoon agave nectar

2 teaspoon kosher salt

Small orange wedge

½ teaspoon chili powder

Directions:

Place 1 teaspoon of salt and chili powder on a plate. Take a glass and pour some orange around its rim.

Blend tequila, lime juice, agave nectar, orange juice, blueberries, and ice cubes until it smoothens.

After blending taste the mixture and add more agave nectar if the taste is harsh. Pour the combination into a glass and put some ice cubes into the glass and serve.

Paloma Cocktail

Preparation time: 5 minutes

Servings: 2

Ingredients:

2 oz. of tequila

2 oz. of grapefruit juice, fresh

2 oz. of water, sparkling

1/2 oz. of lime juice, fresh

1/4 oz. of simple syrup or agave nectar, +/- as desired

For glass rim: sea salt, coarse

For garnishing: grapefruit wedges, fresh

Directions:

Rub grapefruit wedge around the edge. Dip into salt on a small plate.

Mix tequila with sparkling water, grapefruit juice, agave nectar, and lime juice in a glass.

Fill the rest of the glass using ice. Adjust the sweetness, as desired.

Use grapefruit wedge for garnishing and serve.

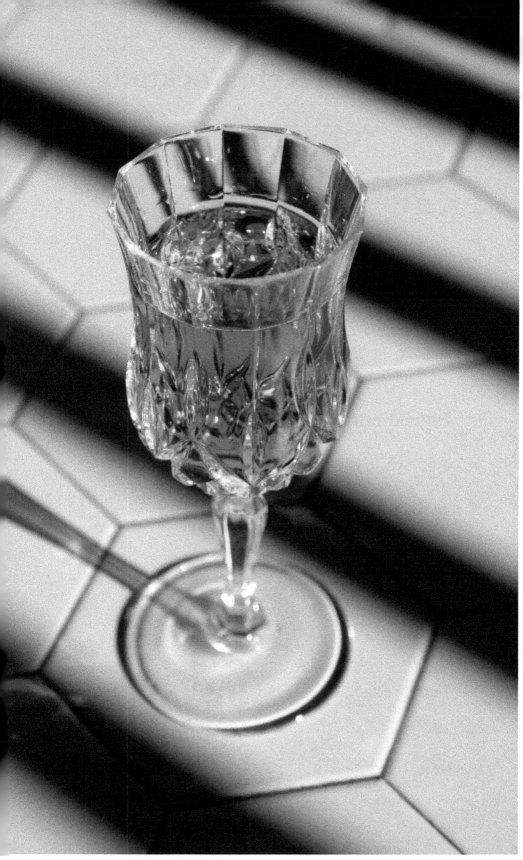

Rum Keto Cocktails

Beachcomber

Preparation time: 10 minutes

Servings: 2

Ingredients:

2 oz. white rum

¾ oz. triple sec liqueur

¼ oz. Maraschino liqueur

¾ oz. lime juice

Ice

Lime wedge, for garnish

Directions:

Pour ¾ oz. of lime juice, ¾ oz. of triple sec liqueur, ¼ oz. of Maraschino liqueur, and 2 oz. of white rum into a shaker

Fill the shaker with ice cubes and shake

Garnish with a lime wedge after straining in a chilled glass

Sweetheart Sunset

Preparation time: 10 minutes

Servings: 2

Ingredients:

10 oz orange juice

2 oz pineapple juice

4 oz light rum

1 tablespoon grenadine

Lime slices, garnish

Directions:

Mix rum and orange juice, combine pineapple juice with grenadine.

Pour orange juice mixture into 2 glasses filled with ice. Slowly pour pineapple mixture on top to create an ombre effect.

Garnish with lime slices.

Cable Car

Preparation time: 5 minutes

Servings: 1

Ingredients:

1½ oz. spiced rum

1 oz. orange curacao liqueur

1 oz. lemon juice

½ oz. sugar syrup

Ice

Orange peel spiral, for garnish

Superfine sugar, for rimming

Directions:

Rim a chilled cocktail glass with sugar

Pour 1 oz. of lemon juice, ½ oz. of sugar syrup, 1 oz. of orange curacao liqueur, and 1½ oz. spiced rum into a shaker

Fill the shaker with ice cubes and shake

Strain into prepared glass

Garnish with orange peel spiral

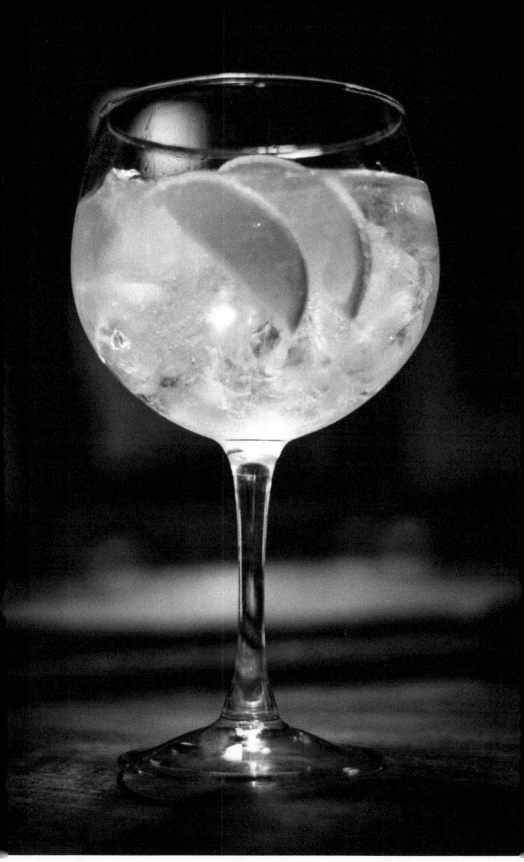

Vodka Keto Cocktails

Perfect Pinot

Preparation time: 5 minutes

Servings: 2

Ingredients:

3 ounces cucumber vodka

1 ounce lemon juice

3 ounces Pinot Grigio wine

2 ounces lemon-lime soda

Ice cubes

4 mint leaves

Directions:

Shake vodka, lemon juice, Pinot Grigio wine, and lemon-lime soda.

Pour into a Collins glass.

Fill with ice cubes.

Garnish with mint leaves.

PinkBerry

Preparation time: 5 minutes

Servings: 2

Ingredients:

3 ounces blueberry vodka

4 ounces lemonade

Ice cubes

3 frozen blueberries

Directions:

Shake vodka and lemonade.

Pour into a Collins glass.

Fill with ice cubes.

Move blueberries to the bottom of a Collins glass.

Fruity Vodka

Preparation time: 10 minutes

Servings: 3

Ingredients:

2 ounces red berry vodka

2 ounces orange juice

2 ounces pineapple juice

1 ounce club soda

Ice cubes

Directions:

Shake red berry vodka, orange juice, pineapple juice, and club soda.

Pour into a Collins glass.

Fill with ice cubes.

Peach Melba

Preparation time: 10 minutes

Servings: 3

Ingredients:

3 ounces peach vodka

1 ounce raspberry syrup

1 scoop vanilla ice cream

Ice cubes

Directions:

Shake vodka, raspberry syrup, and ice cream.

Pour into a Collins glass.

Fill with ice cubes.

Morning Orange

Preparation time: 10 minutes

Servings: 3

Ingredients:

1½ ounces orange vodka

¼ ounce Triple Sec

1 ounce orange juice

3 ounces sweet and sour mix

Ice cubes

Directions:

Shake vodka, Triple Sec, orange juice, and sweet and sour mix.

Pour into a Collins glass.

Fill with ice cubes.

Mucho Melon

Preparation time: 10 minutes

Servings: 1

Ingredients:

1½ ounces cucumber vodka

2 ounces watermelon juice

1 ounce lime juice

4 ounces club soda

Ice cubes

Directions:

Shake vodka, watermelon juice, lime juice, and club soda.

Pour into a Collins glass.

Fill with ice cubes.

Metropolitan

Preparation time: 10 minutes

Servings: 3

Ingredients:

1½ ounces Pomegranate vodka

1 ounce pomegranate juice

1½ ounces grapefruit juice

1 ounce lime juice

Ice cubes

Directions:

Shake Pomegranate vodka, pomegranate juice, grapefruit juice, and lime juice.

Pour into a Collins glass.

Fill with ice cubes.

Ginger Beer Lemonade

Preparation time: 15 minutes

Servings: 4

Ingredients:

1 cup of sugar, granulated

1 cup of water, filtered

6 lemons, juice only, fresh

1 fresh lemon to use for garnishing

8 fl oz. of vodka

2 x 12.7-oz. bottles of beer, ginger

Directions:

Combine filtered water and sugar in a small-sized pot on high heat.

Continuously stir till sugar dissolves and liquid reaches boiling.

Remove mixture from heat. Set aside and allow to cool.

After the mixture cools, add fresh lemon juice. Stir, combining well.

Fill four glasses with ice from filtered water.

Pour 1/4 of the mixture in each iced glass.

Add 2 oz. of vodka to glasses.

Add 6 oz. of ginger beer to glasses.

Use lemon wedges to garnish. Serve.

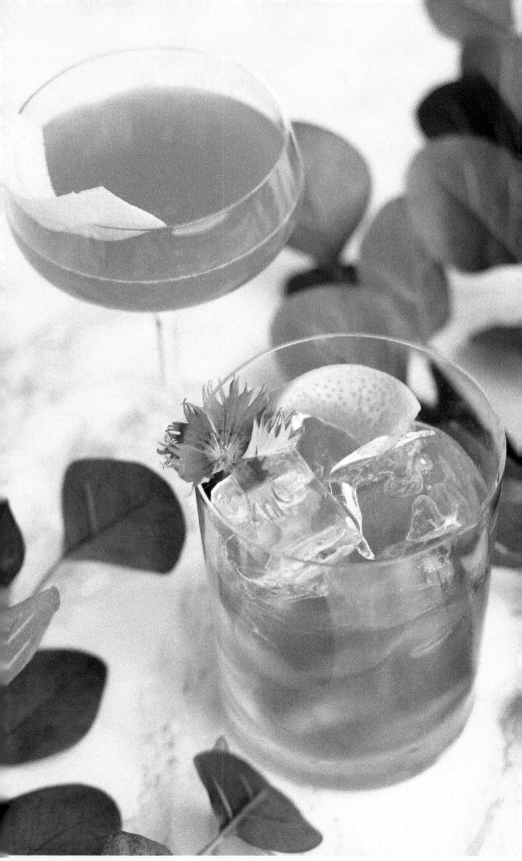

Keto Liqueurs

Safari Juice Recipe

Preparation time: 10 minutes

Servings: 2

Ingredients:

Orange liqueur (30 ml)

Melon liqueur (30 ml)

Orange juice (140 ml)

Grenadine syrup (6 drops)

Directions:

Combine the melon and orange liqueur in a mixing glass and stir.

Add the orange juice and vigorously stir. In a chilled highball glass add ice, then pour in your drink.

Add the six grenadine drops one at a time ensuring not to stir.

Garnish with melon or orange slices.

Purple Devil Recipe

Preparation time: 10 minutes

Servings: 2

Ingredients:

Triple sec (1 part)

Orange liqueur (1 part)

Almond liqueur (1 part)

Cranberry juice

Lemon-lime soda (1 splash)

Directions:

In a cocktail shaker combine the liquors with ice.

Using a highball glass filled with ice, strain the chilled liqueur combo.

Add the cranberry juice to ¾ way up the glass and top off with lemon-lime soda.

Garnish with an orange or lime slice.

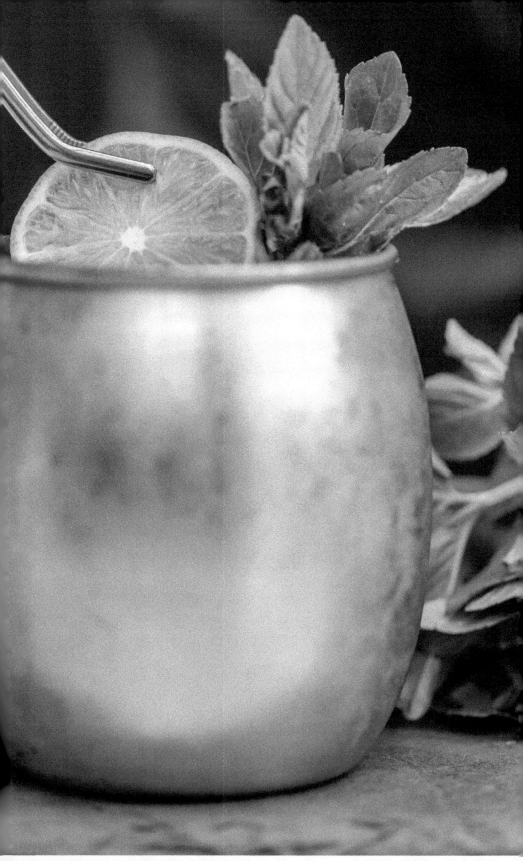

Keto Mocktails

Strawberry Basil Soda

Preparation time: 5 minutes

Servings: 3

Ingredients:

1 lb of strawberries, trimmed

The juice of a half of a lemon

½ of a Cup of loosely packed basil leaves

1 Cup of sugar

Carbonated water

Directions:

Using your knife & cutting board, trim the strawberries.

Place the berries into your blender and process until smooth.

Transfer the berries to the sieve push through using your spatula.

Toss the solids and pour the juice into your measuring cup.

Add sufficient water to fill up the cup.

Put the basil, lemon juice, and sugar into the saucepan.

Place the pan over medium heat.

Cook until boiling.

Reduce the heat and allow the mixture to simmer for five minutes.

Stir often while the mixture is cooking.

Take the pan off of the heat and set it aside to cool.

Pour the syrup mixture through the sieve into your container.

Toss solids.

Now spoon two Tbsp of the syrup into your glass.

Pour carbonated water on top & stir.

Serve and enjoy.

Lemonade Mojito Mocktail

Preparation time: 5 minutes

Servings: 3

Ingredients:

4 oz of Lemonade

4 oz of Sprite or 7UP

1 oz of mint mojito syrup

1 mint sprig

Directions:

Place enough ice in your glass to fill it halfway.

Add all of the ingredients & stir.

Use a mint sprig as garnish.

Virgin Mojitos

Preparation time: 5 minutes

Servings: 3

Ingredients:

2 Cups of water

1 & ½ of Cups of white sugar

2 Cups of chopped mint leaves, chopped

2 Cups of lime sherbet, softened

1 Cup of lime juice

1 Cup of water

8 Cups of club soda

1 Lime

Directions:

Begin by slicing the lime & chopping the mint leaves.

Now place the water & sugar into the microwavable bowl.

Place in the microwave and cook on high for five minutes.

Now the mint leaves into the water and stir.

Allow the mixture to sit for five minutes.

Run the mixture through your sieve.

Toss the leaves and set the mixture aside.

Put the sherbet, a Cup of water & lime juice into your picture.

Stir until the mixture is thoroughly combined.

Now add that mint syrup into the mixture.

Add in the club soda & stir.

This drink should be served over ice.

Use lime slices for garnish.

Coffee Ginger and Marmalade Mocktail

Preparation time: 15 minutes

Servings: 3

Ingredients:

Ginger Syrup:

1 ounce fresh ginger (peeled, and thinly sliced)

½ cup water

½ cup sugar

Mocktail:

¼ cup freshly-brewed espresso

1 tbsp ginger syrup

1 tsp Seville orange marmalade

Ice

1 orange twist (to garnish)

Directions:

For the ginger syrup: In a small pan, combine the fresh ginger with water and sugar. Simmer until the sugar entirely dissolves.

Cover with a lid and steep for 20 minutes.

Strain the syrup into a mason jar and allow it to cool.

Use as directed, and store any leftover syrup in the fridge for up to 28 days.

For the **Mocktail:** Add the espresso, ginger syrup, and marmalade to a cocktail shaker filled with ice, and shake it all about.

Strain into a coupe glass and decorate with a twist of orange.

Sherbet Spider

Preparation time: 65 minutes

Servings: 3

Ingredients:

1 cup of cranberry juice

1 cup of soda water

Fresh mint

2 cups of Greek yogurt

1 ½ cups of buttermilk

2 tablespoons of fresh lime juice–lime slices to serve

3 cups of frozen raspberries

1 cup of icing sugar

1 teaspoon of vanilla extract

Directions:

Into a saucepan over a low flame, combine raspberries, icing, vanilla, and 1 tablespoon of lime juice.

Let it cool.

Pour in buttermilk and yogurt.

Pour into a jug with a lid.

Into the freezer till frozen.

Spoon into Glasses.

Top with cranberry, lime, and soda water.

Place mint on top to serve...

Orange Mango Crush

Preparation time: 10 minutes

Servings: 3

Ingredients:

2 cups of orange juice

2 cups of mango nectar–chilled

4 scoops of lemon sorbet

2 cups of soda water–chilled

Ice

Orange slices

Directions:

In a blender, blitz orange juice and sorbet.

Pour into a jug.

Add soda and nectar.

Stir well.

Pour over ice and orange slices.

Pine banana mocktail

Preparation time: 10 minutes

Servings: 3

Ingredients:

Pineapple Pieces: 2 oz.

Bananas: 2

Sugar: 1 oz.

Pineapple Juice: 4 oz.

Sprite: 4 oz.

Ice as required

Directions:

Cut the pineapple pieces and put them in a blender jug.

Add in the banana pieces and pineapple juice.

Blend it well to make a smooth drink.

Add in sugar and blend again.

Take the serving glass and put ice in it.

Fill the glass with the drink you have made.

Top with sprite and serve.

Slushy espresso

Preparation time:1 hour 40 minutes

Servings: 3

Ingredients:

Espresso: 4 oz.

Sugar: ¾ oz.

Lemon Juice: ¼ oz.

Lemon Zest: ¼ oz.

Cream: 1 oz.

Water: 4 oz.

Directions:

Take a saucepan and add water and sugar to it.

Bring to boil.

Remove from the heat and add espresso to it.

Strain the liquid in a bowl and let it rest until cool.

Add in the lemon juice and lemon zest.

Add this liquid to a shallow dish and put it into the freezer.

Take this out every 30 minutes, crush the mixture, and put it again in the fridge. (3 cycles)

When done, put into the serving glass and garnish with cream.

White choco mocktail

Preparation time: 10 minutes

Servings: 3

Ingredients:

Passion Fruit: 2 (halved)

Peach: 1 (chopped)

Coconut Water: 4 oz.

Caster Sugar: 1 oz.

White Chocolate: 2 oz.

Vanilla Extract: ½ oz.

Coconut Cream: 1 oz.

Ice as required

Directions:

Remove the passion fruit skin and put it in a bowl. Discard the seeds.

In a blender jug, add peaches, the pulp of the fruit, coconut water, and sugar: blend well to make a smooth puree.

Take a pan and heat it super hot.

Add in chocolate, cream, and vanilla extract.

Stir and cook until the mixture is done.

Take your serving glass and add some ice to it.

Add in the puree and top with the chocolate mixture.

Serve it and enjoy.

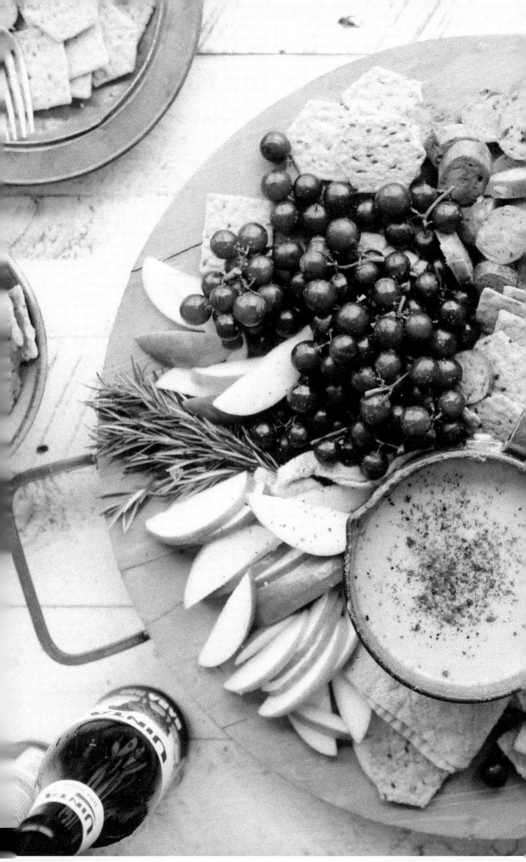

Keto Snacks for Happy Hour

Salmon and CherryTomatoes Salad

Preparation time: 5 minutes

Cooking Time: 5 minutes

Servings: 4

Ingredients:

3 oz. smoked salmon

½ oz. leafy greens

½ oz. cherry tomatoes

½ oz. red bell peppers

½ oz. cucumber

¼ scallion

3 tablespoons mayonnaise

Directions:

In a bowl add all ingredients and mix well. Serve with dressing

Nutrition: calories 260, fat 8, fiber 2, carbs 8, protein 35

Antipasto Salad

Preparation time: 5 minutes

Cooking Time: 5 minutes

Servings: 4

Ingredients:

12 oz. romaine lettuce

3 tablespoon parsley

4 oz. mozzarella cheese

3 oz. ham

3 oz. salami

4 oz. canned artichokes

2 oz. roasted red peppers

1 oz. sun-dried tomatoes

2 tablespoons olives

½ cup basil

1 red chili pepper

¼ tablespoon salt

Directions:

In a bowl add all ingredients and mix well. Serve with dressing

Nutrition: calories 260, fat 8, fiber 2, carbs 8, protein 35

Keto Avocado and bacon Salad

Preparation time: 5 minutes

Cooking Time: 5 minutes

Servings: 4

Ingredients:

8 oz. cheese

6 oz. bacon

2 avocados

3 oz. walnuts

3 oz. arugula lettuce

Dressing

¼ lemon

¼ cup mayonnaise

¼ cup olive oil

1 tablespoon heavy cream

Directions:

In a bowl add all ingredients and mix well. Serve with dressing

Nutrition: calories 340, fat 1, fiber 2, carbs 8, protein 22

Pastrami Salad with Croutons

Preparation time: 5 minutes

Cooking Time: 15 minutes

Servings: 4

Ingredients:

1 cup mayonnaise

1 tablespoon mustard

1 shallot

1 dill pickle

6 oz. lettuce

9 oz. pastrami

4 eggs

6 low-carb parmesan croutons

Directions:

In a bowl add all ingredients and mix well. Serve with dressing.

Nutrition: calories 340, fat 1, fiber 2, carbs 8, protein 22

Keto chaffle with ice-cream

Preparation time: 5 min

Cooking Time: 5 min

Servings: 2

Ingredients:

1 egg

1/2 cup cheddar cheese, shredded

1 tbsp. Almond flour ½ tsp. Baking powder.

For serving

1/2 cup heavy cream

1 tbsp. Keto chocolate chips.

2 oz. Raspberries 2 oz. Blueberries

Directions:

Preheat your mini waffle maker according to the manufacturer's instructions. Mix chaffle ingredients in a small bowl and make 2 mini chaffles.

For an ice cream ball, mix cream and chocolate chips in a bowl and pour this mixture into 2 silicone molds.

Freeze the ice cream balls in a freezer for about 2-4 hours.

For serving, set an ice cream ball on the chaffle.

Top with berries and enjoy!

Nutrition: calories 100, fat 7, fiber 2, carbs 8, protein 6

Walnuts low-carb chaffles

Preparation time: 10 minutes

Cooking Time: 20 minutes

Servings: 4

Ingredients:

2 tbsps. Cream cheese

½ tsp almonds flour

¼ tsp. Baking powder

1 large egg

¼ cup chopped walnuts

Pinch of stevia extract powder

Directions:

Preheat your waffle maker.

Spray waffle maker with Cooking spray.

In a bowl, add cream cheese, almond flour, baking powder, egg, walnuts, and stevia.

Mix all ingredients,

Spoon walnut batter in the waffle maker and cook for about 2-3 minutes.

Let chaffles cool at room temperature before serving.

Nutrition: calories 275, fat 20, fiber 2, carbs 8, protein 20

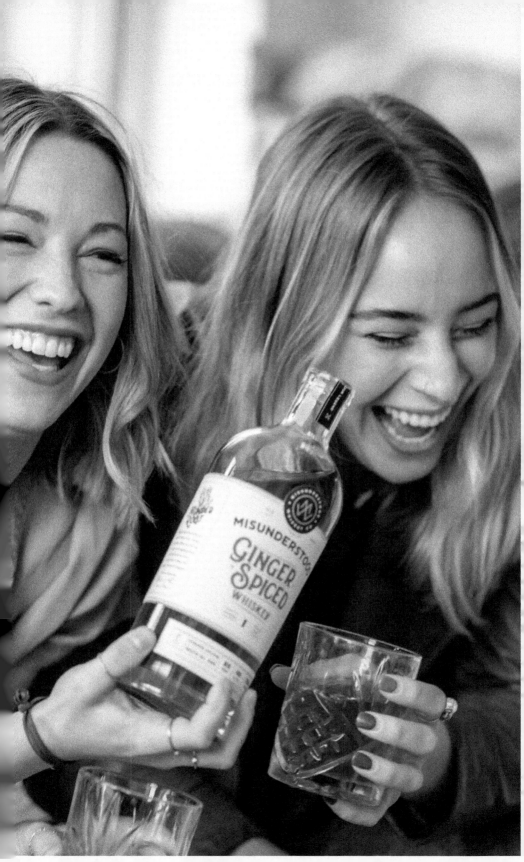

Conclusion

Here we come to the end of our keto cocktail journey. Each unique cocktail has a specific recipe, although you can vary some ingredients to taste. You should taste every component of your drinks if you do them right. Perfect drinks are balanced between sour and sweet flavors. Outside of sweet and fruity drinks and those with chocolate, your cocktails will usually be somewhere between sweet and sour. I hope my cocktails have helped you improve your lifestyle.

Lightning Source UK Ltd.
Milton Keynes UK
UKHW021948140621
385519UK00002B/423

9 781802 895797